# EMPOWERED WOMEN
# Helping Others

## Great Advice from the Front Lines of Life

Carole Hale Bishop
John Bishop

**FOX PUBLISHING**

## DEDICATION

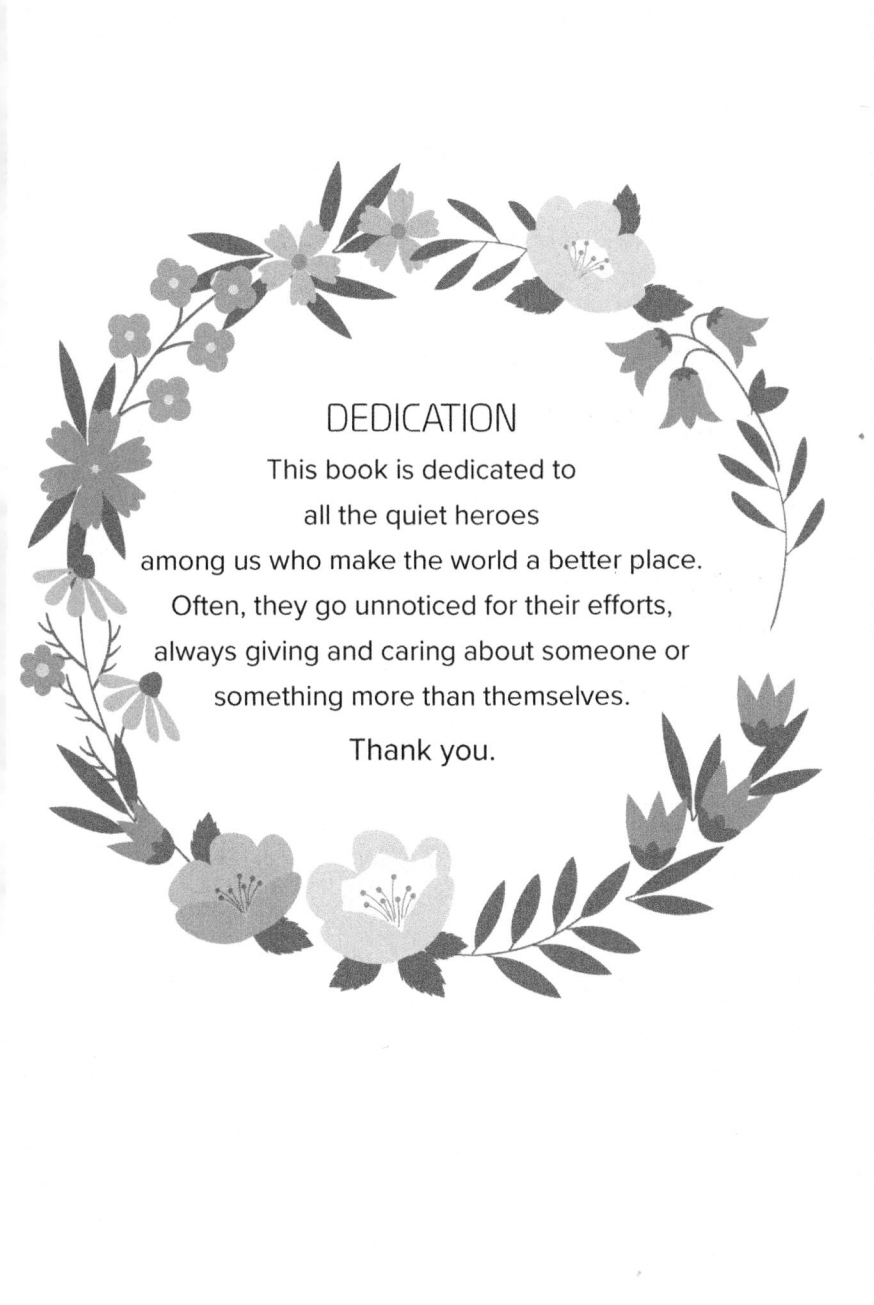

This book is dedicated to
all the quiet heroes
among us who make the world a better place.
Often, they go unnoticed for their efforts,
always giving and caring about someone or
something more than themselves.

Thank you.

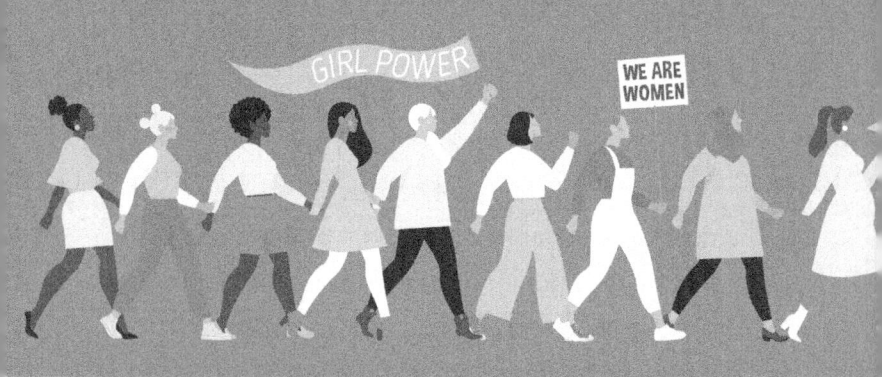

Published by Fox Publishing

Copyright @ 2020 Carole Hale-Bishop & John Bishop

All rights reserved. No part of this publication may be reproduced, stored in a retrieval system, or transmitted, in any form or by any means, electric, mechanical, photocopy, recording, or otherwise, without the prior written permission of Bishop & Company, LLC. The exception is in case of brief quotations embodied in critical articles or reviews.

**Contact Information**
Carole Hale – Bishop
John Bishop
www.TeachingMoments.com

## BOOK CONTENTS

The book is designed for personal reflection, journaling, and open discussion with others.

1. The Desiderata
2. Life Lessons
    a) 24 Gold Coins
    b) Wants – Needs – Desires
    c) 10 Things Anger Steals from You
    d) Confidence Builder
    e) Two Great Questions to Ask Each Day
    f) 10 Roadblocks to Success
    g) Five Scariest Words
    h) Bummer Words
    i) 10 Rules About Money
    j) 10 Life Lessons Learned on a Unicycle
    k) 10 Ways to Prepare for Success
3. Two "Advice from Other Cultures" sections
4. Four License Plate Ideas
5. Two "You Are Not Alone" sections
6. Three Descriptive Words
7. Your Turn

# INTRODUCTION

We asked hundreds of women, just like you, one question:

**What is the Best Advice You Ever Received?**

Many women submitted their advice and life lessons in hopes of making your journey a little easier, more rewarding, and hopefully, a little more fun. This is the first in a series of self help books.

The **Empowered Women Helping Others** book is about helping you navigate this crazy, complicated, fun, exciting, sometimes scary world we live in.

**The book includes:**

- 225 + easy-to-implement tips on self-esteem, raising kids, working, single parenting, dealing with midlife crisis, overcoming obstacles, stress management, reducing fear and much more.
- Top 10 Roadblocks to Your Success
- Two "You're Not Alone" sections
- Two Great Questions to Ask Yourself Everyday

- 10 Rules About Money
- 10 Ways to Prepare for Success
- Multiple areas for reflection and places to journal

**FREE book:**

For upcoming books, we are looking for people willing to share their life lessons to help others. If we use your advice, we will send you a free copy of the book as a thank you gift. See www.teachingmoments.com/advice.

Your journey may include a myriad of challenges such as single parenting, midlife crisis, loss, self-confidence, divorce, Parkinson's Disease or Autism, etc. Your problems might seem overwhelming at times, but you are not alone. People sharing their life experiences will remind you that there is light at the end of the tunnel. You are a winner!

- **NOTE:** A portion of each sale will go to the Michael J. Fox Parkinson's Foundation and autism research. Thank you.

**Contact Information**
Carole Hale – Bishop
John Bishop
www.teachingmoments.com

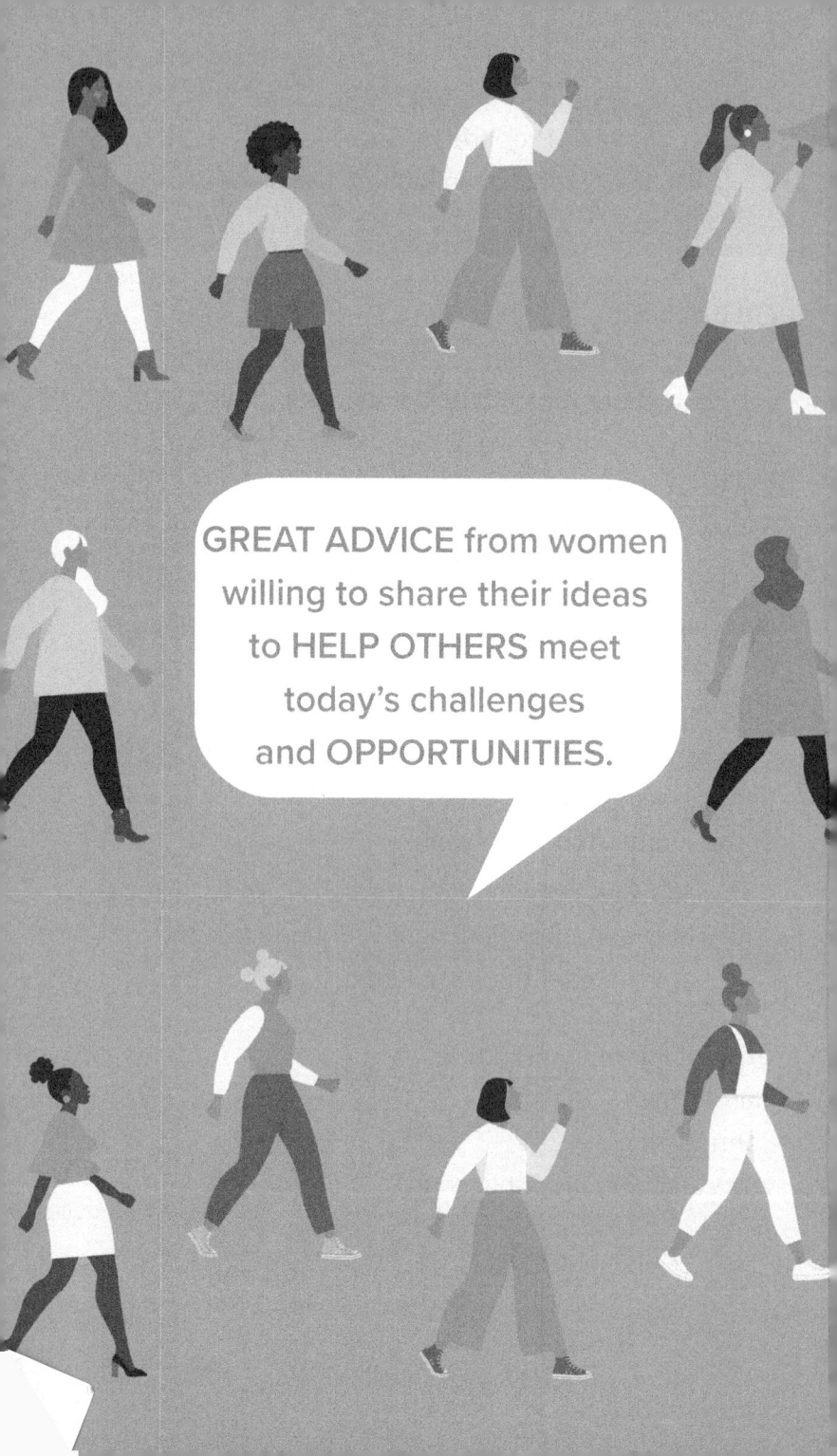

GREAT ADVICE from women willing to share their ideas to HELP OTHERS meet today's challenges and OPPORTUNITIES.

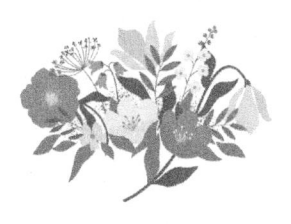

## THE DESIDERATA

Go placidly amid the noise and haste and remember what peace there may be in silence.

As far as possible, without surrender, be on good terms with all persons. Speak your truth quietly and clearly; and listen to others, even to the dull and the ignorant, they too have their story. Avoid loud and aggressive persons, they are vexations to the spirit.

If you compare yourself with others, you may become vain and bitter; for always there will be greater and lesser persons than yourself. Enjoy your achievements as well as your plans. Keep interested in your own career, however humble; it is a real possession in the changing fortunes of time.

Exercise caution in your business affairs, for the world is full of trickery. But let this not blind you to what virtue there is; many persons strive for high ideals, and everywhere life is full of heroism. Be yourself. Especially, do not feign affection. Neither be cynical about love, for in the face of all aridity and disenchantment it is perennial as the grass.

Take kindly to the counsel of the years, gracefully surrendering the things of youth. Nurture strength of spirit to shield you in sudden misfortune. But do not distress yourself with imaginings. Many fears are born of fatigue and loneliness.

Beyond a wholesome discipline, be gentle with yourself. You are a child of the universe, no less than the trees and the stars; you have a right to be here. And whether it is clear to you, no doubt the universe is unfolding as it should.

Therefore, be at peace with God, whatever you conceive Him to be, and whatever your labors and aspirations, in the noisy confusion of life, keep peace in your soul.

With all its sham, drudgery, and broken dreams, it is still a beautiful world.

Be cheerful. Strive to be happy.

*Leann S., submitted this poem from Max Ehrmann*

### Stash the Memories

Take the time to soak in the experience, be it a major event or even just hanging out with friends. Stash the memories away!

*Heather P.*

### Footprints

Everything in life has repercussions; be proud of the footprints you leave behind.

*Nicole S.*

## Love Who You Are

".... love yourself...love who YOU are and be the best YOU".

Teenagers struggle so much with finding themselves and being accepted by their peers. If we teach them self-love...it'll all work itself out. ...a second piece of advice would be the Golden Rule... treat others as you want to be treated. That rule is priceless!

*Sara E., advice from a mother*

## Someone Else Will

Make a plan for yourself or someone else will do it for you.

*Laura C.*

## Three R's

Respect myself
Respect that others have their story
Take Responsibility for all your actions.

*Kay T*

## Burning Bridges

Don't burn your bridges . . . you never know when you might need them.

*John M., advice from his dad*

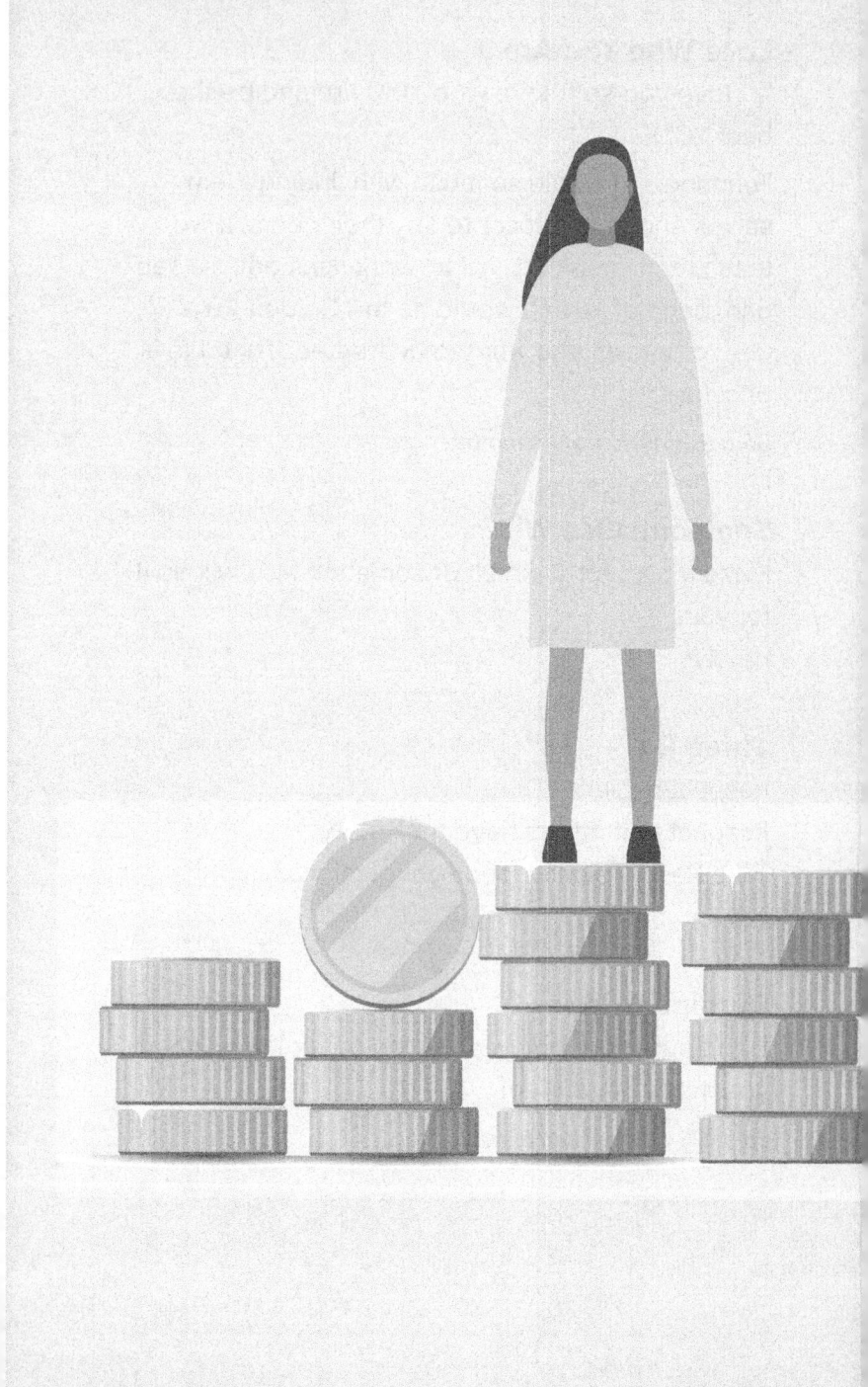

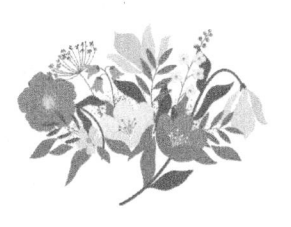

## 24 GOLD COINS

A man I knew was given six months to live, yet his outlook on life was inspiring.

I asked how he could stay so positive knowing he only had a short time to live. He shared these thoughts with me.

"Each day when I wake up, I receive twenty-four gold coins, one for each hour of the day. I spend some of those coins for eating, sleeping, time with my family, and taking care of the day's responsibilities. I choose to spend some of my daily hours (coins) having fun and helping others. At the end of each day there are usually a couple of special gold coins left over. I spend these with particular care."

What an invaluable life lesson for us and our children. We live in a hectic, "there is never enough time to get everything done" world. Our future success, and that of our children, will be determined by how wisely we invest our daily gold coins.

How would you spend your special gold coins? Some suggestions:

- Help a child with their homework.

- Start a project that you have "been meaning to get to."
- Spend thirty minutes a day learning something new.

### Enjoy Life

Always do the right thing. Do something fun every day.

Live each day as if it were your last. Enjoy life!

*Sofía L.*

### Thirsty

Dig the well, before you are thirsty.

*Bella A.*

### Top Priority

Integrity should be a top priority.

*Lisa B.*

### Build a Better You

"...God said to build a better world. And I asked how.....

And  God .....said just build a better you."

*Kris H.*

### Consequences

You can do whatever you want to do....if you are willing to pay the consequences.

*Jenni P.*

### Life Decisions

Know what you believe and why you believe it.

*Valentina W.*

## { QUOTE FOR DISCUSSION }

Children will do what you do, not what you say.

*Neil W.*

Your thoughts

### Negotiating
When you are negotiating, ask them what they WANT; most of the time it will be a lot less than what you were thinking of giving."

*Bella B., advice from her dad*

### Share Your Thoughts
Show people what you want, and what you are willing to do to get it. Share your thoughts with people and you will discover there are plenty of people to help you.

*Julie R., advice from her mother*

### Job Skills
In your current job build skills you will use in your next job.

*Tina G.*

### Wisdom
Arrogance is never a positive. Self-confidence is.

*Martha G.*

### Commitment
Always finish what you start. Fulfill your commitment.

*Evelyn C.*

# LICENSE PLATE IDEA

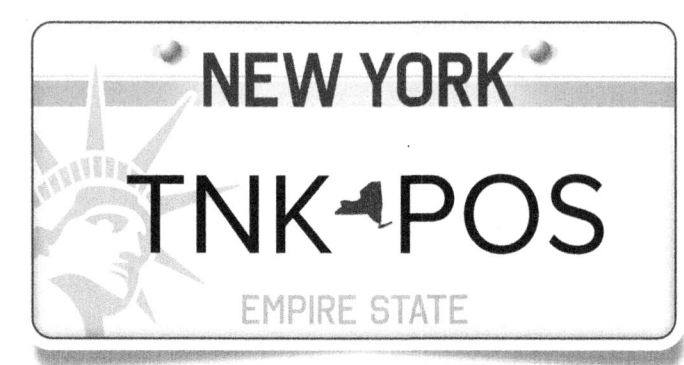

**NEW YORK**
**TNK POS**
EMPIRE STATE

The license plate will be a daily reminder for you, and it may help others.

### Unto others
Do unto others as you want them to do unto you.
*Kaiulani G., submitted this Bible verse*

### Art of Business
Good business is always a win-win.
*Gretchen U.*

### 3 Words
Less is more.
*Joshua E.*

### Can't Outrun Your Past?
You cannot outrun your past!
*Alma C.*

## Core Values
Know your core values.

*Kana G.*

## Check Your Ego
Put your ego in your back pocket.

*Luciana L.*

## Only Way to Success
There is only one way to succeed - performance, performance—every time.

*Acari*

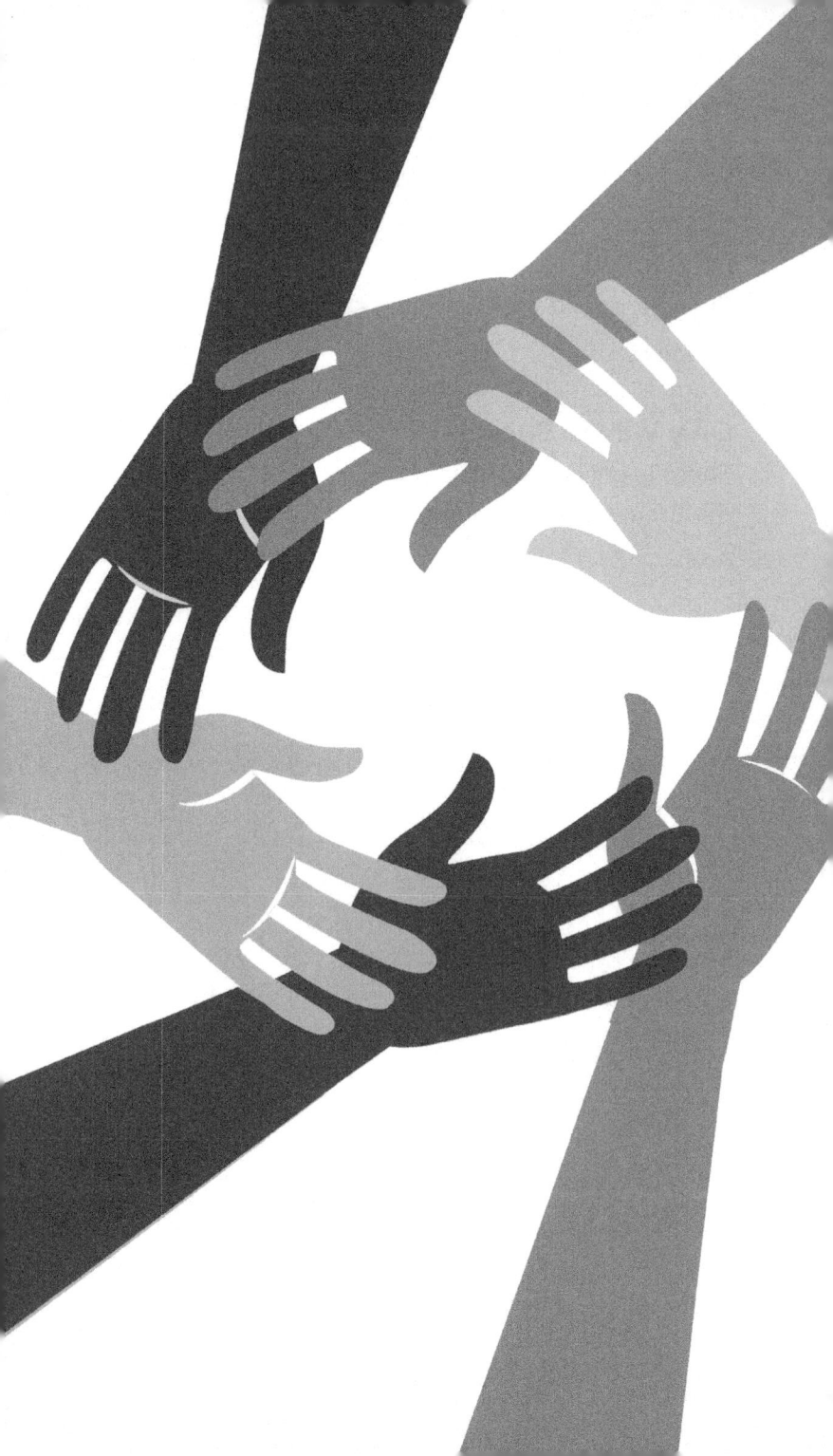

# WANTS – NEEDS - DESIRES

We all live in a rapidly paced world where success is often defined by the "bigger, better, faster" aspects of life i.e., bigger house, faster car, better golf score, etc. That is the "rat race" most of us profess to despise. Did you know that you can control your level of involvement in it? The control switches are your wants, needs and desires.

### Needs

Abraham Maslow, a noted professor of Psychology, theorized that people have five basic needs, i.e., shelter, food, security (which can include the security of employment, money, health, religion), love/belonging (friendship, family, work groups, clubs, religious groups), and respect (a feeling of self-esteem, valued for our thoughts and ideas).

### Wants

Wants help us to improve ourselves in one or more of the five basic needs categories: I want a better job; I want to get an "A" on the next history exam; I want to start exercising to improve my health, etc. However, wants without a plan are simply wishes. To change "wants" into success stories you need to develop a plan that includes a goal, action steps and a timetable for completion.

### Desire

Desire is the fuel that ignites your passion. This is the most powerful of the three control switches because it directly impacts the other two. Desire has the power to change imagination into reality, doubt into risk-taking, fear of change into motivation and roadblocks into minor setbacks. Your desire, your passion, is what excites you and prepares you to meet the day's challenges.

### Suggestions for implementation:

- Write down two examples of your "needs." Be specific.
- Write down one example of your "wants."
- Write down the one "desire." What propels you each day and gives you the energy to face the day enthusiastically?
- Which of the examples can you build a plan around to accomplish something new?

_____
_____
_____
_____
_____
_____
_____
_____

## Your Customer's Business

Your business grows with the growth of your customer's business. Help them grow.

*Renee D.*

## My Decisions = My Success

Success depends on me making good choices.

*Jennifer W.*

## Self-Inflicted Wounds

Most of one's wounds are self-inflicted.

*Michelle W.*

## Help

Help is in front of you if you look.

*Yui K., advice from a college professor*

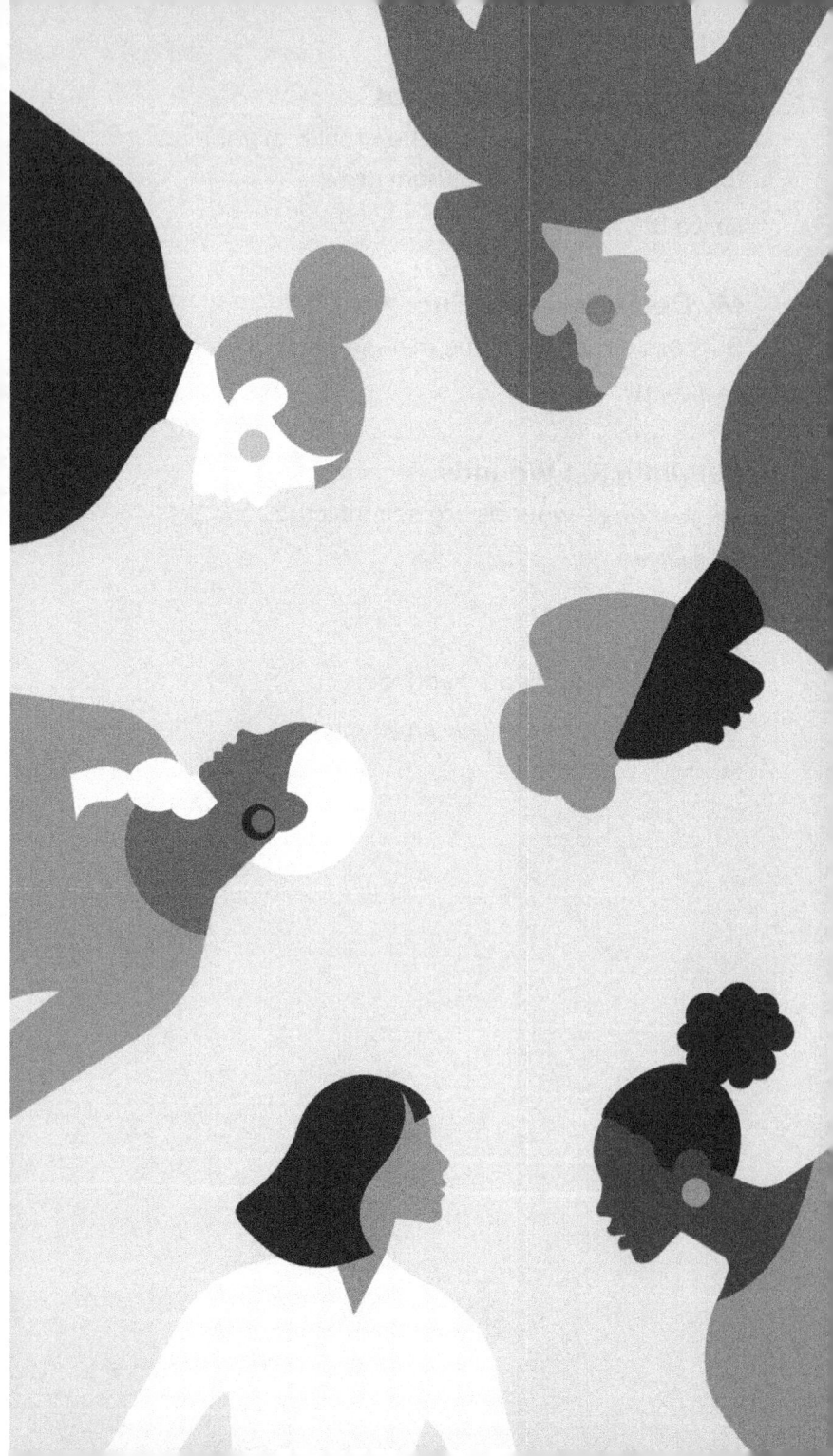

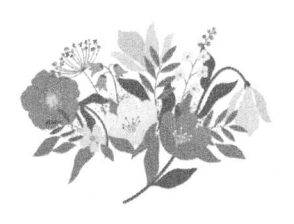

## 10 THINGS ANGER STEALS FROM YOU

Anger is a natural emotion that each of us experiences. When used correctly it can motivate us into action to complete a task or right an injustice. This type of anger can give us a strong sense of accomplishment when we take immediate action to correct the injustice or perceived wrong.

However, anger can also be a thief. When someone directs anger negatively toward themselves or others, anger steals from that person.

**10 Things Anger Steals from You:**

1. Anger can steal your time.
2. Anger can steal your energy.
3. Anger can steal your self-respect.
4. Anger can steal your relationships with family, friends, and co-workers.
5. Anger can steal your ability to communicate effectively.
6. Anger can steal your sense of right and wrong.
7. Anger can steal your vision of the future.

8. Anger can steal your health.
9. Anger can steal your sense of well-being.
10. Anger can steal your problem-solving skills.

If you do not control your anger, it will control you. Uncontrolled anger is giving your personal power to someone else. An important part of life is learning how to effectively deal with anger issues. Anger can be a positive motivator or a powerful negative influence. Ultimately, it is your choice.

**Can you relate to one or more things anger was stolen from you?**

_____
_____
_____
_____
_____
_____
_____
_____
_____
_____
_____
_____
_____
_____
_____
_____

### Earn More
To earn more - read more, learn more, do more.

*Elizabeth M.*

### Preparation
You will only go as high as your five (5) closest friends.

*Carol M., advice from a friend*

### Advice from the Front Lines
Listen to the people on the front lines. They usually have valuable first-hand information. Been there, done that.

*Donna G.*

### Do Your Best
They always told me to do my best at everything.

*Camille P., referring to her parents*

### Unreasonable Man
"A reasonable man adapts himself to his environment. An unreasonable man persists in attempting to adapt his environment to suit himself. Therefore, all progress depends on the unreasonable man."

*Cindy C., submitted this quote by George Bernard Shaw*

### Don't Jump
Don't jump to conclusions. Too often you will be wrong.

*Alexandra F.*

### Kids Need Reminding
Teach your kids how to make positive, healthy decisions and the importance of helping others.

*Janice H.*

### The Small Stuff
Don't sweat the small stuff... and remember it is all small stuff.

*Suzi S. (this is also the title of an excellent book)*

### Eliminate Fear
Be who you want to be - not who others think you should be.

*Kesha F., advice from her Dad*

## {QUOTE FOR DISCUSSION}

Network with EVERYONE. Treat ALL people with respect. The person you meet today may greatly influence your life sometime in the future.

*Scott H.*

Your thoughts

_____
_____
_____
_____

## Self-Growth
Helping others helps you.

*Ami S.*

## Stand Up for What You Believe
"To thine own self be true..."

*Teresa M., quote from Shakespeare*

## Preparation
If you fail to prepare, then prepare to fail.

*Darleen W., quote from Ben Franklin*

## Single Parenting
Single parenting is like the person trying to spin five plates on narrow dowels. If you get all the plates spinning at a time, it can be rewarding. But, have one fall and it can be devastating.

*Fiona O.*

## Enjoy What You Can
Enjoy what you can and remember that every action can have an unequal and completely opposite reaction.

*Darcy M.*

## Trust and Truth
"He who does not trust enough, will not be trusted."

*Mindi, J., quote from Lao Tzu.*

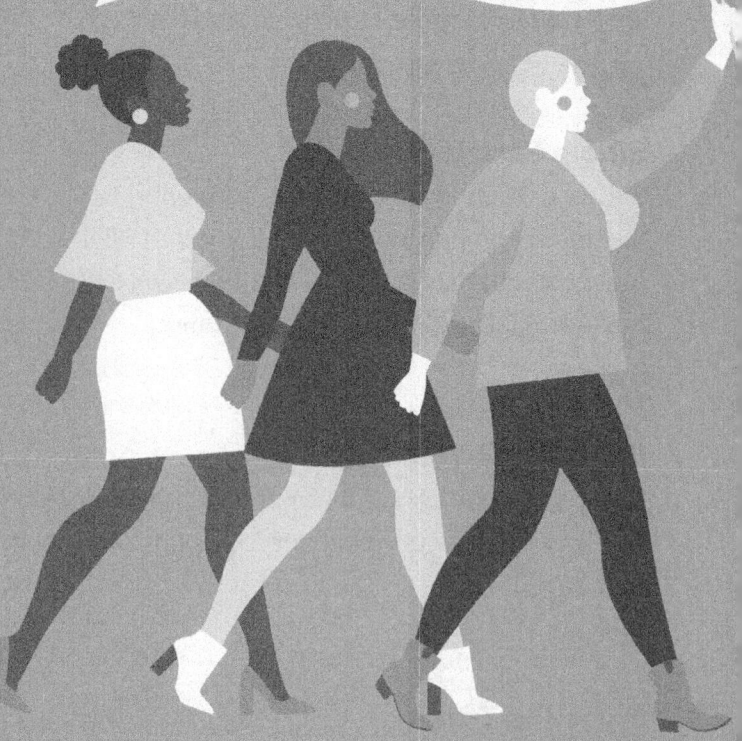

SUCCESS

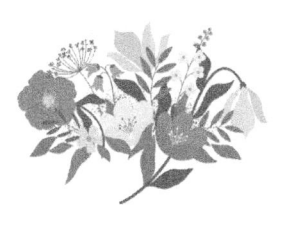

## **CONFIDENCE BUILDER**

"Always Leave it on a Good Note"

My husband used this life lesson with our grandson, and it has had a big impact on how Kyle sees himself as an athlete. Hope the idea will help you.

When Kyle was seven or eight, John would take him to the YMCA to shoot baskets. Probably only 25% of the shots went in, but Kyle loved playing basketball. But, at some point John would say "it's time to go. Shoot one more basket." John let Kyle shoot and shoot and shoot until he made a basket for his last shot. As they walked off the court, John would say: "Always leave on a good note."

Why was that last shot so important? Because it is the one, he will remember. He walked of the basketball court a winner. That is what he remembered. Even today, when Kyle is doing something important, John will say "leave it on a good note."

How can you use this confidence building idea?

## Dressed in Overalls

Sometimes opportunity comes dressed in overalls and looks like work.

*Jeannie F., advice from her father, a quote from Thomas Edison*

## Risk

Never underestimate the value of taking a risk on yourself. It's the best risk you can take. Don't let anyone tell you otherwise.

*Roshini R.*

## Who?

Know who you are.

Like who you are.

Be who you are.

*Tamara V.*

## Be Confident

Listen and learn with your eyes and ears.

*Teresa A.*

## No Limitations

Don't ever let anyone tell you what your limitations are, you never know until you try. Never stop dreaming.

*Carole S.*

### Everyone Else
Be yourself, everyone else is taken.

*Janna A., quote from Oscar Wilde*

### Change
God, grant me the serenity to accept the things I cannot change, the courage to change the things I can,
and the wisdom to know the difference. Amen

*Kerri P., submitted the Serenity Prayer*

# { QUOTE FOR DISCUSSION }

## Changing Victim Mentality

"…. no matter what happens in our life that we cannot control, we can always control our response to what happens."

Victor Frankl, who was a survivor of a Nazi war camp, said that choice is the greatest human freedom. When you work with difficult people, or when the stock market crashes, or when you suffer from inevitable disappointments, realize you have the power as to how to act and that the "victim mentality" rarely leads to success.

*Jennifer C., supplied this quote from Victor Frankl*

How do you deal with change, stress, or choice?

### Job Perspective

Keep your job in perspective. You can be replaced at any time. Be flexible.

*Ebony H.*

### Suffering

Suffering is optional.

*Elizabeth L.*

### Revolving World

The world doesn't revolve around you, so get over yourself.

*Barb K., advice from a youth minister*

### Walk and Talk

Walk the walk, not talk the talk.

*Kaiulani G., lesson learned from Girl Scouts*

### Help Others

You can have everything in life that you want if you will just help enough other people get what they want.

*Aiysha S., quote from motivational speaker Zig Ziglar*

### Feeling Lonely

I called home feeling lonely. My mom said, "no one will knock on your door when they don't know where you live."

Translation....network, network, network

*Sandra B., advice from her mother*

## Knife in the Back

Be careful. The knife you stick in someone's back today, may be attached to your new boss tomorrow.

*Margaret, advice from her dad*

# HELPING OTHERS

1. **Do you have some advice you want to share?**

   This book is the first in a series. If we use your advice, we will send you a free copy when the book is published. www.TeachingMoments.com/advice

2. **Write a review.**

   Most people looking for a book go to the Amazon's Customer Reviews section to see what others thought of the book. Your review of **Empowered Women Helping Others** will help others make their decision. Note: Please look for "ratings section" on the book's Amazon's page and write a review.

3. **Tell a friend.**

   If this book helped you, maybe it will help someone you know and care about. The Tell-A-Friend form is in the middle of the website's home page. ww.teachingmoments.com.

   Thank you for helping others.

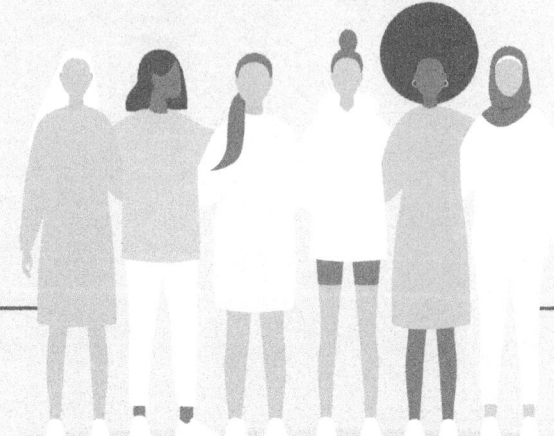

**LOOK FOR OTHER BOOKS COMING IN 2021**

## YOU ARE NOT ALONE

Famous People who have overcome disabilities

- Thomas Jefferson, U.S. President, dyslexia
- Princess Diana, Princess of Wales, depression
- Tiger Woods, golfer, stuttered when he was young
- Abe Lincoln, US President, bipolar disorder
- Tom Cruise, actor, dyslexia
- Walt Disney, co-founder of Disney, ADHD
- Christopher Reeve, actor, wheelchair bound
- Ben Stiller, actor, bipolar disorder
- Davis Beckham, soccer, obsessive compulsive disorder
- Kristi Yamaguchi, Olympic champion, club foot

**Dip Your Toe**

You can never dip your toe in the same spot in the river—ever changing, ever evolving...be able to change with it.

*Sandy K.*

## What's Next
Do what's next. Simple advice but accurate.
*Nancy C.*

## Visions of Grandeur
All youth have visions of grandeur...don't become another statistic.
*Bonnie W.*

## Harder and Smarter
The harder and smarter you work - the luckier you get.
*Liz M., quote from Gary Player, Hall of Fame golfer*

## Extra 30 Minutes
Show up to work at least 30 minutes early and stay 15 minutes more than required.

If you want a career instead of simply a job, this is a good way to get noticed. After that, it's how well you perform. Good luck.
*Shelia H., advice from a career advisor*

# TWO GREAT QUESTIONS

Ben Franklin was the 15th child of a poor family and had only three years of formal training. Yet, he overcame many potential obstacles to forge a successful life for himself and contribute to his country. During his 84 years he became an author, publisher, inventor of the lightning rod and the Franklin stove, one of America's Founding Fathers, signed the Declaration of Independence, and was the United States Ambassador to France. Mr. Franklin was a lifelong learner who taught himself five languages and could play several musical instruments.

Ben Franklin lived a rich and full life by developing some strong personal character traits. For example: Two Great Questions

1. When he started the day he asked, "What good will I do today?
2. Before bed he asked, "What good did I do today?"

**This is a simple, easy to do and compelling life lesson from one of our country's founding fathers.**

How would your life change if you daily started asking these two questions?

_____
_____
_____
_____

### Dress Rehearsal

Life is not a dress rehearsal. Mistakes are part of learning and growing. Be positive and helpful to others. This is a "WE" world not an "I" world.

*Latanya B., advice from a teacher*

### If it Stinks

If it stinks, it's rotten.

*Alexa K.*

### Look at Yourself in the Mirror

If you can't get up in the morning and look at yourself in the mirror, smile and say "I'm glad to be going to work today" it's time to find a new job!

*Andrea T., advice from a former boss*

### Two Life Questions

What do you want out of life, and how hard are you willing to work to get it?

*Junaid W.*

## Who Gets Credit

It's amazing what you can achieve when you let go of your ego. Don't let your ego get in the way of a good decision.

*Miranda P.*

Yes, I Can, I WILL

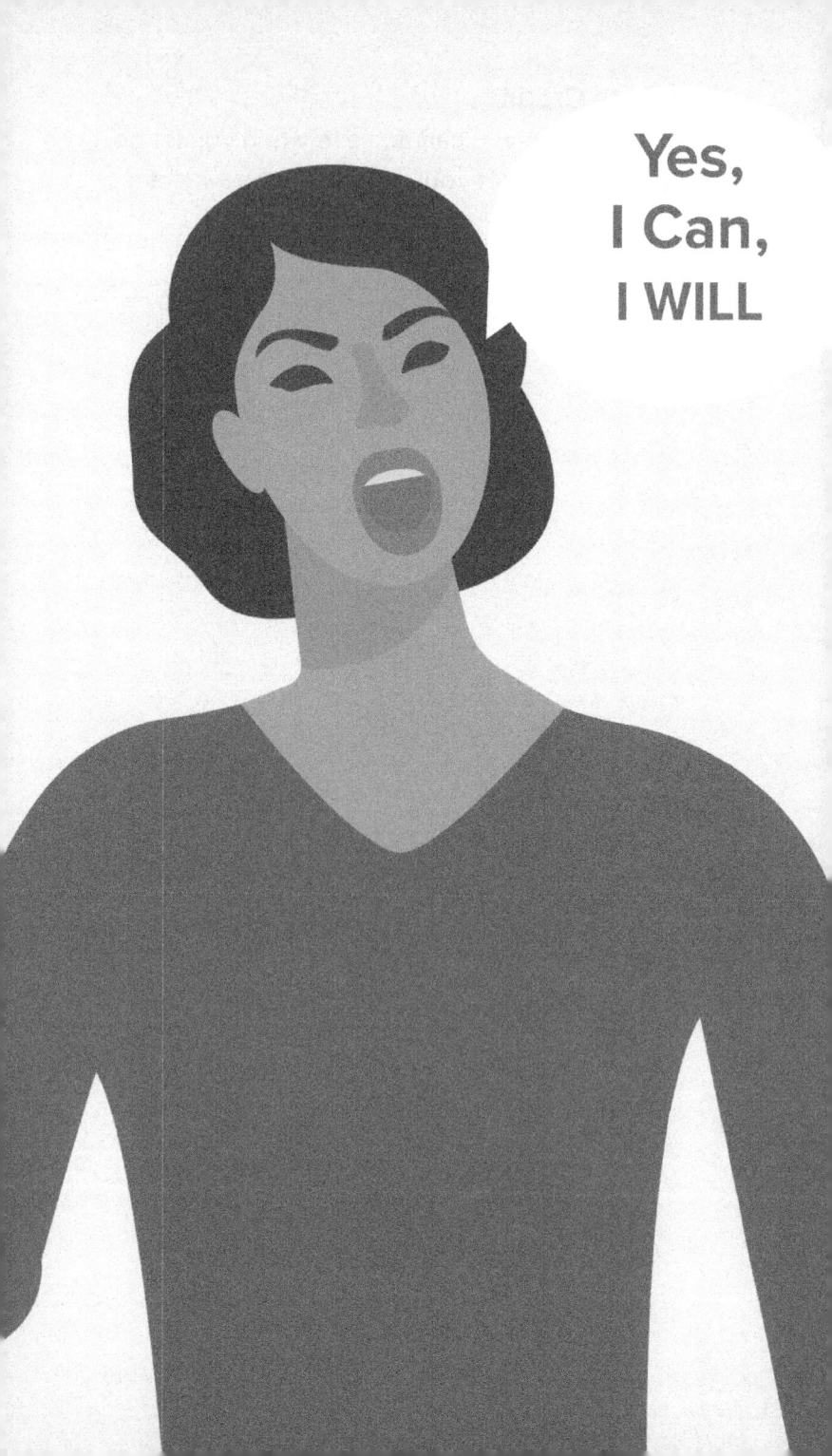

# THE 5 SCARIEST WORDS

The 5 scariest words in the English language are: yes, I will, and *I can*. Why? Because as soon as you say them you have made a commitment.

**For example:**

- Yes, I will help at the church fish fry on Saturday.
- Yes, I can make the decorations for the wedding.
- I will take that new job.

Depending on your level of commitment, these five words can also be you're "I'll Make It Happen" words.

_____
_____
_____
_____
_____
_____
_____
_____

### Gambling

In gambling and in life there are three choices: win, lose or draw. It's always your choice.

*Helen C.*

### The Worst That Can Happen

What's the worst that can happen, you fail? Remember you can't fail if you don't try.

*Shelley W., advice from her mother*

### Get and Education

Get an education and have a Plan B.

*Marge D., advice from her grandmother*

### Measure It

If you can measure it, you can make it better.

*Michelle M.*

### Forget the Rest

Set the objective and then break it down to realistic action steps.

*Lashawn B.*

### Learn-Share-Find-Know

Learn about other people. Find the good in everybody. Be a realistic dreamer.

*Sara R.*

### Commitments vs. Excuses

Winners make commitments and losers make

excuses.

*Lucia., advice from her minister, quote from John Schuerholz, Baseball Hale of Fame*

## Slowdown and Think
Measure twice. Cut once.

*Janet M.*

## Key to Failure
Trying to please everybody.

*Stefani J.*

## Learn to Sell
Life is selling yourself, your ideas, products, and services. Learn how to sell.

*Isabella F.*

## Stick to It
Once you make a commitment, stick with it! Be realistic. Start small and build on your successes.

*Elizabeth R.*

## Reality
Don't sell yourself short.

*Raegan B.*

## It's Up to You
If it is to be, it's up to me.

*Sandy K.*

### Assumptions
Never assume.

*Janice D.*

### What's Right is Right
Do the right thing because it is the right thing to do.

*Alison C., quote from Martin Luther King*

## { QUOTE FOR DISCUSSION }

### Stealing your day

Don't let anyone steal your good day. If someone or something interrupts your good day, deal positively with the situation. Don't let it wreck the rest of your day.

*Jessica H.*

Your thoughts?

_____
_____
_____
_____
_____
_____
_____
_____
_____

## First Impressions

Be ready to create a good first impression. Yes, you can't judge a book by its cover, but first impressions are especially important.

*Helena B.*

## What Follows

Always strive to do your best. The rest will follow.

*Ellyn J.*

### Karma

Karma's a bitch. Everything you give out comes back to you.

The good AND the bad. Be kind.

*Anita D.*

# {QUOTE FOR DISCUSSION}

If you had to give a friend one piece of advice about relationships, what would it be?

## Selling

Ask for the order! After you get it, stop talking and leave. Many sales are lost by too much talking after the sale.

*Andrea O., advice from her sales manager*

## Speak Less

Listen more than you speak.

*Yvonne S.*

## Moving Forward

When you stop learning you stop moving forward. The world is filled with stuck-in-their-old-way-of-thinking people. Continue learning and growing.

*Jackie W.*

## It's Too Hard

It's never too hard if you are ready to sacrifice enough. Hard work, focus, and a mental positive attitude will get you ahead. Helping others will keep you there.

*Heather I.*

## Forgiveness

It's easier to beg for forgiveness than ask for permission.

*Kathy J.*

### Weight Loss

I've found that you can't lose weight if you are not happy.

*Gretchen H.*

### Can't Control

"I don't worry about what I can't control."

*Amanda W. supplied this quote from Miami Dolphins Coach Don Shula after a poorly officiated game*

# LICENSE PLATE IDEA

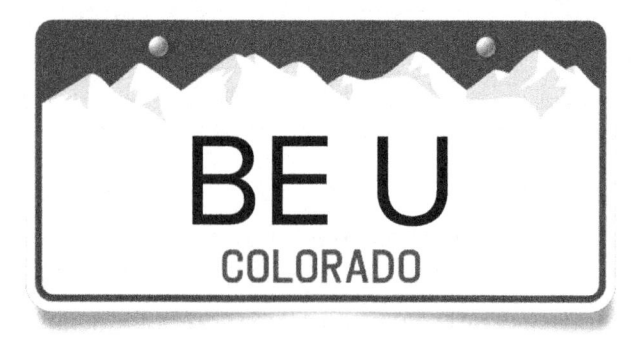

The license plate will be a daily reminder for you, and it may help others.

### Ask for Help

Do not be afraid to ask for help. You'll be amazed by what you can accomplish.

*Emma B.*

### Take a Detour

For every failure, there's a lesson.

You just have to find it.

Failure can be a gift if you learn, change, and grow from it.

*Suri S.*

### Win and Loss

It is important to learn how to win and lose. Both build character.

*Elizabeth R.*

### A Belt and Suspenders

Never trust a man wearing a belt and suspenders. He doesn't even trust himself.

*Francis F.*

### Listen Well

Chart your own path. Be grateful. Ask for help. Be kind. Help others. Listen well. Only positive self-talk.

*Shauna F.*

## {QUOTE FOR DISCUSSION}

### Peer Pressure

Peer pressure is doing something that a group or individual wants you to do, even if you are reluctant to do so.

How has positive or negatively peer pressure affected your life? Has it been your motivation or your boat anchor?

## Living Life Correctly

Be respectful. Act respectful. Earn respect.

*Jasmine F., advice from her mother*

## Don't Wait - Row

Don't wait for your ship to come in. Row out to meet it.

*Brittany S.*

## Plan for Your Future Success

Plan for the worst, hope for the best.

*Lindsay T.*

## Listening

There are two types of listeners:

1. One listens to learn.
2. The other listens for an opening so they can express their views on the subject. Which one are you? Are you losing important opportunities to learn something new?

*Jessica S.*

### Networking

Network, network, network. Treat everyone with the same amount of respect. Learn from others. Help others.

*Jackie T.*

### Find a Mentor

Find a mentor. Someone who has been there/done that and can give you wise council. This applies to everything – work, relationships, money, sports, etc.

*Kelly G.*

### Smart Parents

The older you get the smarter your parents will become.

*Jessica A.*

### Credit Card

They are not your friend. Get rid of all but one. If you can't pay for it, you probably don't need it. Use a credit card wisely.

*Kris K.*

### Bird in the Hand

A bird in the hand is better than two in the bush. Sometimes, just be happy with what you have.

*Patricia C.*

## Small Children
You can tell a lot about a person if you watch how they treat children and animals.

*Jasper T.*

## Fear
Never fear failure.

*Helen G.*

## Nightly Review
A question before bed: Did I make my life or someone else's better today?

*Charlotte A.*

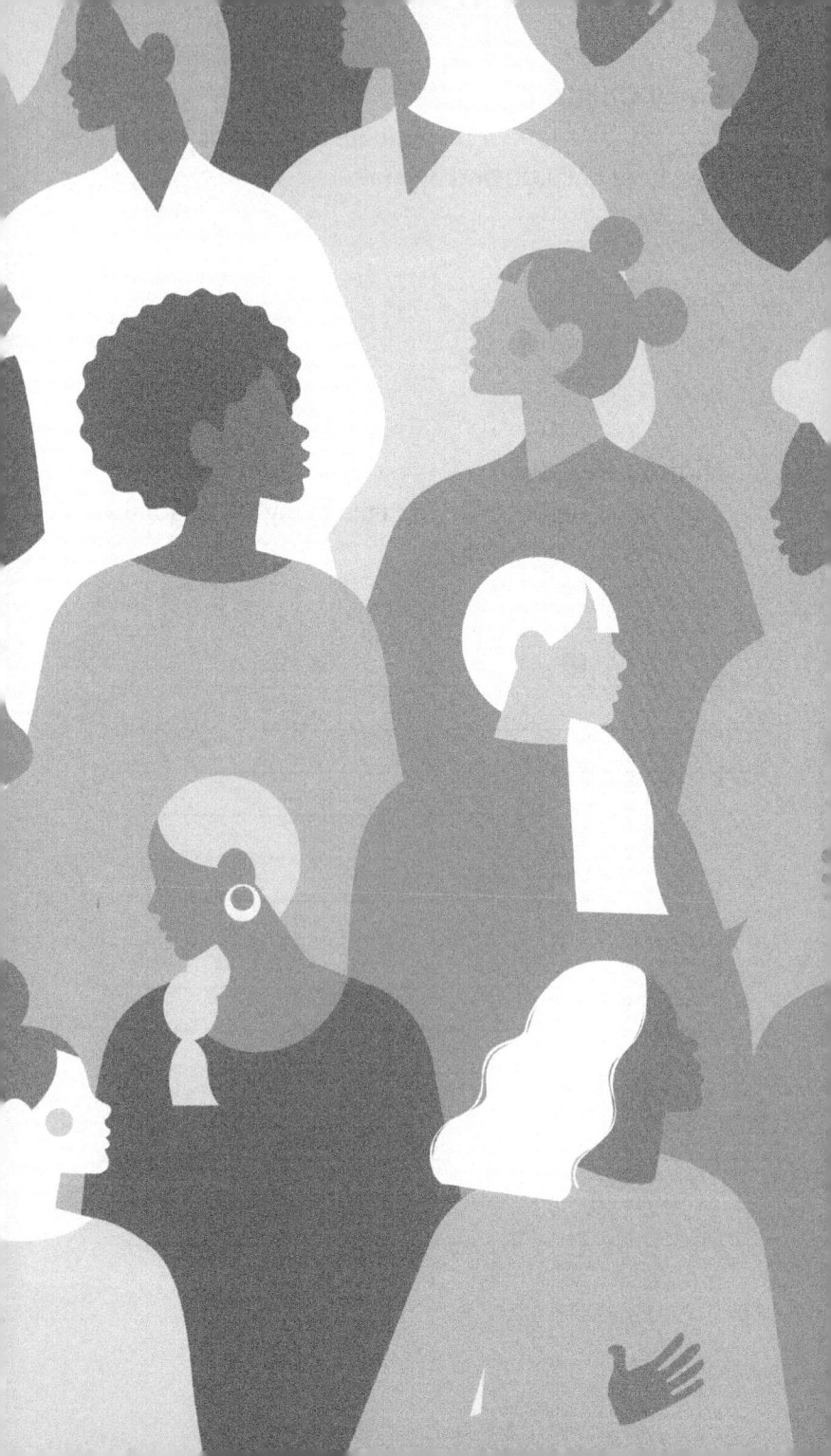

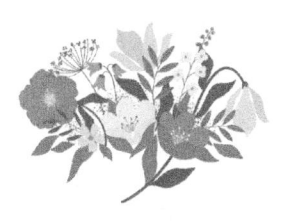

## 3 DESCRIPTIVE WORDS

In three words, how would your friends describe you?

_____,

_____,

_____

Do you agree with them? _____

### Never a Liar
Lying hurts you more than then telling the truth.
*Jackie S.*

### Slow Down & Think
Turn off the cell phone and the iPod; shut down the computer. We lived without them for years. Be resourceful. Find time for nature. Get off the couch and take a walk. Find time to restore your batteries.
*Gretchen W.*

### Short Words – Big Meaning
Ten two letter words — if it is to be, it is up to me
*Razi D.*

### No Put Downs
Don't let others put you down. Most time they are just jealous. Dream big and go for it.
*Camile G.*

### Not Fair
"Life is not fair. Be a Team Player. Be grateful for your blessings.
*Margie G.*

### No Upside, Only Downside
Thirty—three percent of your day is at work. Enjoy it or at least like it or find something else. Life is too short to waste 1/3 of your life on something you

don't like. Find something that uses your talents, with people who appreciate your efforts. Smile, you are loved.

*Annette G.*

## Who You Know?
It's not what you know, but who you know. Make sure people you know, know what you know. It will open many doors.

*Latonya A., advice from her father*

## The Big Three
Health, Family, Work, God, Friends. Have balance in your life.

*Ricki G.*

## Pigs
Do not wrestle with Pigs (read stupid people). Two things can happen:

1. You will get dirty
2. The Pig will enjoy it.

*Patricia J.*

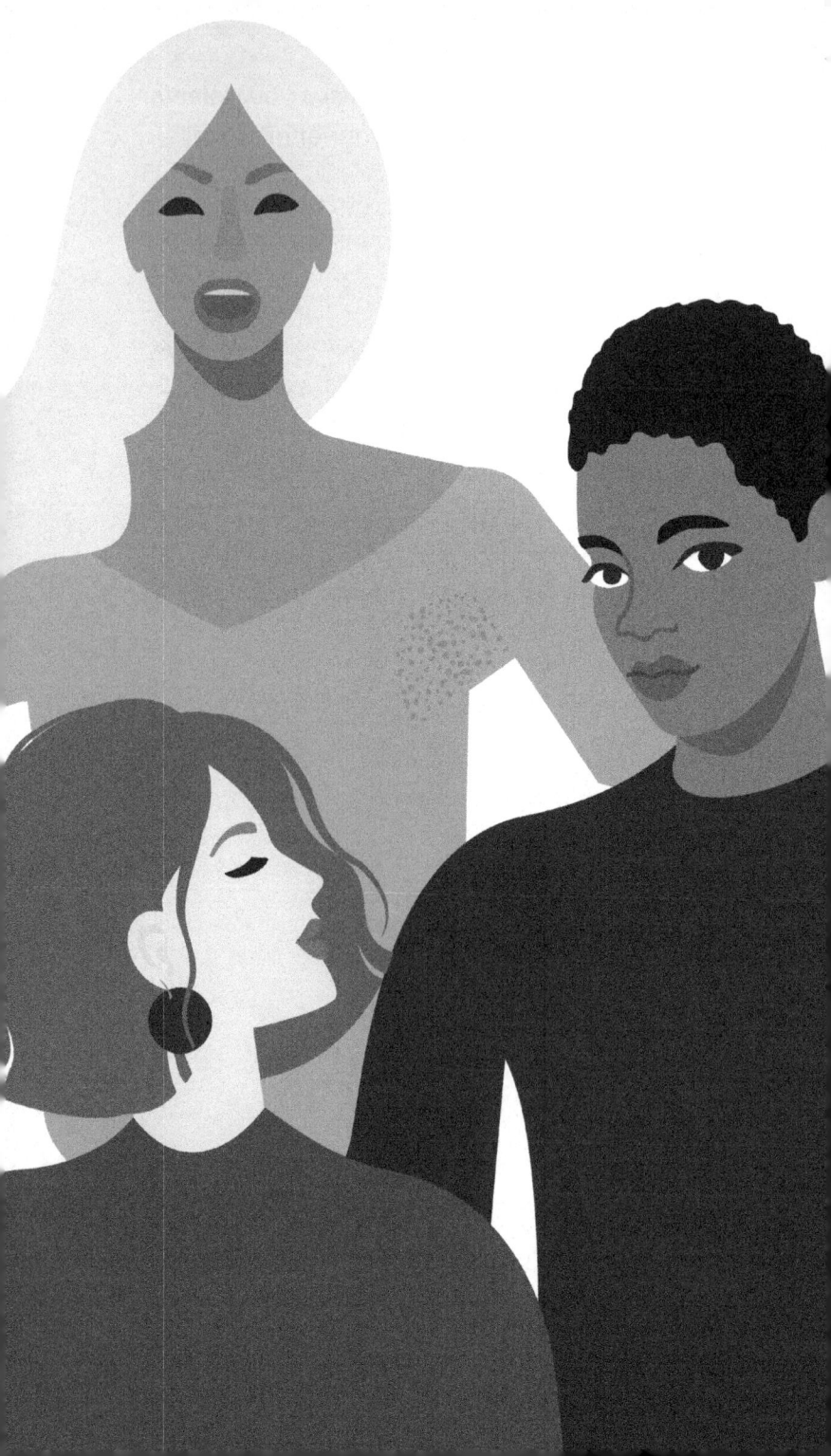

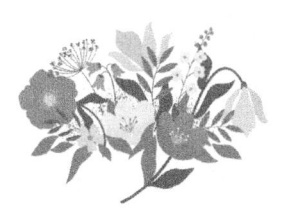

# TOP 10 ROADBLOCKS TO YOUR SUCCESS

Life can seem like a roller coaster at times with plenty of ups and downs. Your success will be determined by how well you meet various challenges along the way. Here are ten potential roadblocks and potential responses for your success.

1. **No clear vision**
   - The clearer your vision the faster you will achieve it. Visualize yourself reaching your goal and enjoying the success – however you define it.

2. **Fear of failure**
   - Do not let worry, fear and uncertainty hold you back from reaching your full
   - potential. Eliminate the Bummer Words - no, never, can't, won't, maybe and if.
   - Ask for help.

3. **Lack of determination**
   - Turn challenges into opportunities to grow. Don't let a challenge become a stopping point on your path to success. Sometimes it takes

more grit and willpower.

4. **No action plan**
   - Talk is cheap — action pays the bills. Write a step-by-step plan of action. Include your vision, action steps and a timetable for completion. Now place the written strategy where you can read it, every day.

5. **Negative thinking**
   - Everyone has some self-doubt and negative self-talk. The good news is that you control the on - off switch. When having negative thoughts, ask yourself two questions: 1) Did I give my best effort to today's activities? 2) Did I help others today?

6. **Change**
   - You will have to make adjustments in your life. Be flexible but remain focused on your goal. Get back on track or find a new path to accomplish your goal.

7. **Lack of enthusiasm**
   - All days are good; some are better than others. You can gain enthusiasm in many ways from successfully completing a task, trying something new or conquering a fear. Be the day's cheerleader. You will find enthusiasm is contagious; give some to others.

8. **Procrastination**
   - As the Chinese say: A journey starts with a

single step. You can have the best plan in the world, but if you don't act on it, you only have a dream. Are self-motivated, or do you need motivation from someone else? Determine which method of motivation works for you. Take action and don't be afraid to ask for help.

9. **Making excuses**
   - Take personal responsibility for your success by eliminating excuses. Avoid blaming others for your lack of effort. Remember the two questions from #5 - Negative Thinking.

10. **Learn from your mistakes**
    - Everyone makes them. Successful people learn extremely valuable life lessons from their mistakes. You learn more about yourself from failures than from your **success**.

These roadblocks can be steppingstones and learning experiences on your life's journey. *YOU ARE A WINNER!*

Which of these roadblocks seems to cause you the most problems? How can you change that area into something more positive for you?

_____
_____
_____
_____
_____
_____
_____
_____

## Seven Jobs

You will likely have 7 - 10 jobs in your career. After each job, take some time to write down what you learned, what you liked, what you didn't like, what type of manager motivates you and the real reason you left the job. Set up a file to keep these notes from your various jobs. It will help you focus on your career development.

*Nacelle M, advice from a career counselor*

## Be Amazed

You will be amazed how many people will quickly help you if asked. If they turn you down, consider yourself lucky. You didn't need their help anyway.

*Amanda R., advice from her father*

## Self-Critique

Think beyond today. Self-critique but do it positively. If you goofed up – learn.

*Altair J.*

## Competitive Advantage

Read.

*Sami F.*

## Mark Twain is Right

"Always do right. This will gratify some people and astonish the rest".

*Lashawn W., submitted this quote from Mark Twain*

## Scary Things

No matter how scary it looks, try. Just be smart about your choices.

*Martha M., advice from her mom*

## Control Worry

Worry about the things within your control, and not the things you cannot control.

*Denise A.*

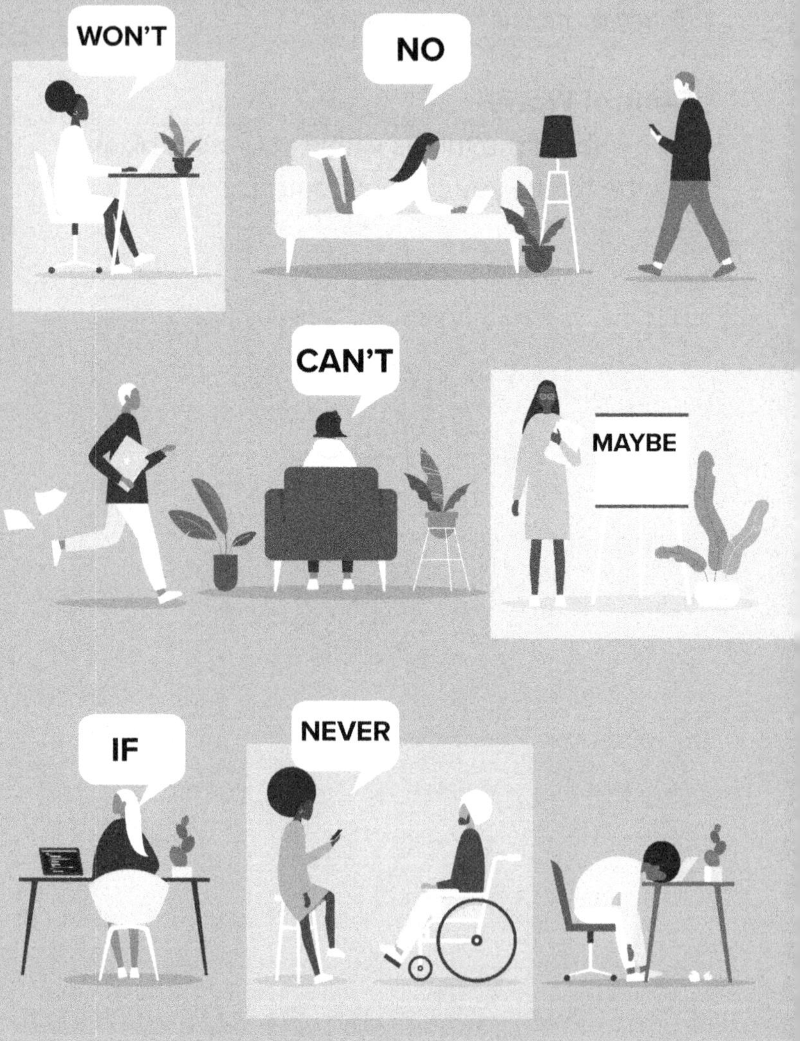
WON'T
NO
CAN'T
MAYBE
IF
NEVER

## BUMMER WORDS

Did you know there are words we use every day that can hold us back from reaching our full potential? We call them the Bummer Words - **no, can't, won't, never, if** and **maybe.** These six words can top us before we even get started on a new task .

Certainly, there are many times where it is appropriate to use these words. As adults we know there are times when it is necessary to use these words. For example: No, I won't get into the car because you have been drinking.

They become **Bummer Words** when we use them as an excuse for not doing something that will challenge us or stretch our capabilities. For example:

- "I'll never get a good grade on that test."
- "I'll try it, but I won't be any good."
- "I won't get that promotion."

**Suggestions for implementation:**

- For the next couple of days, count the num-

ber of times you use one of the six Bummer words.
- Resolve to use one less **Bummer Word** each day.
- Replace them with the positive "I'll Make It Happen" words: *yes, I can*, and *I will*.

___

### Look Inside
Your vision will become clear only when you look into your heart. Who looks outside, dreams. Who looks inside, awakens.

*Jessica M. submitted this quote from Carl Jung, psychologist*

### Good Leaders
A good leader surrounds themselves with great people. Then, gives them room to grow.

*Sandy K.*

## You're #1

Good news: You are the most important in the world.

*Bad news: The person next to you also thinks the world revolves around them.*

Lesson: Neither one of you are correct. Learn to get along with others

*Camille N.*

## Resistance

Persistence beats resistance!

*Rachael V.*

## Youth is No Excuse

There will always be people who say that you are too young to do things. Go out there and prove them wrong. Don't forget to ask for help and to help others.

*Julie R., advice from her teacher*

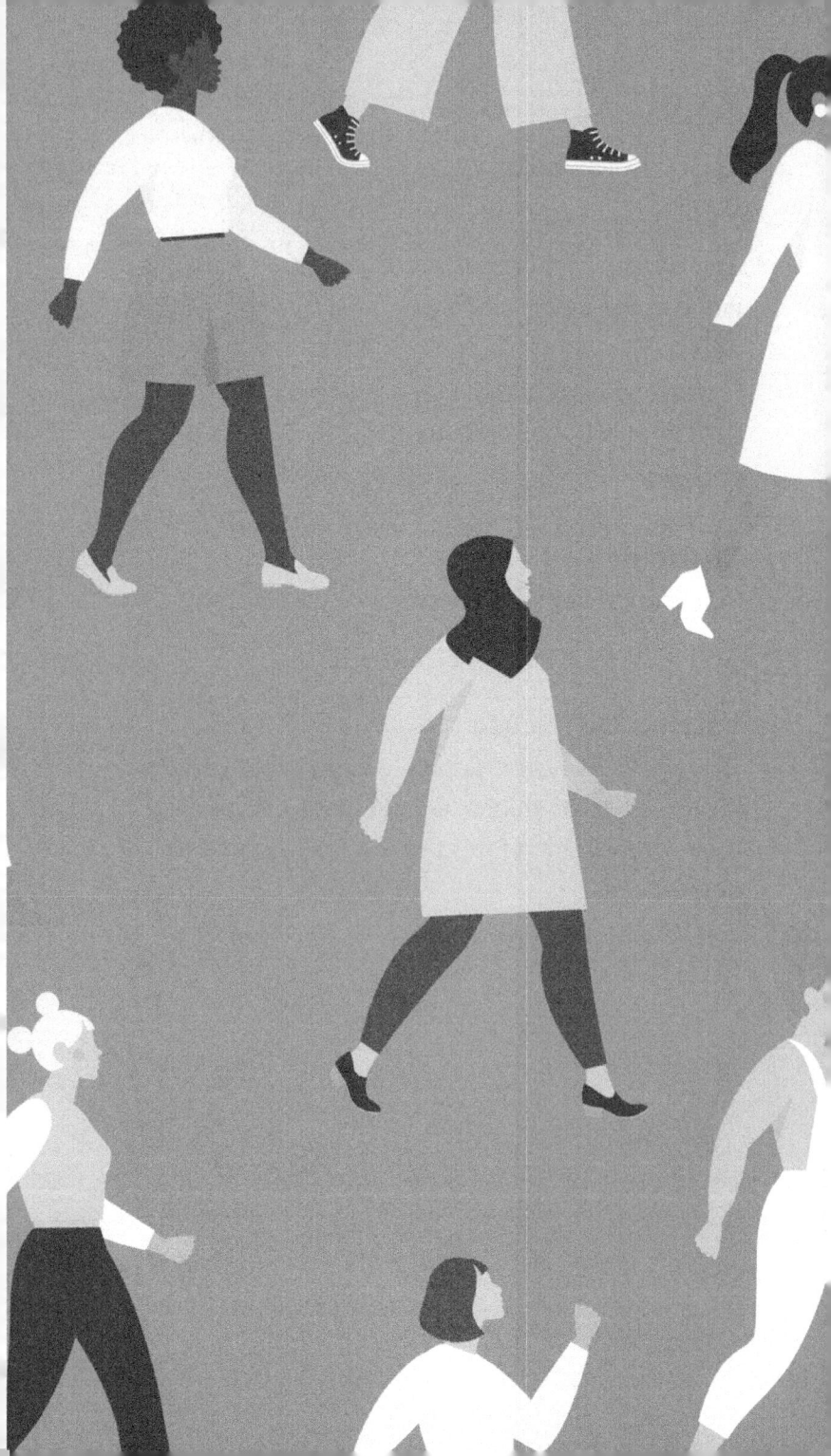

# **YOU ARE NOT ALONE**

Famous people who have overcome disabilities

- Michael Jackson, singer, obsessive compulsive disorder
- Payton Manning, football, cleft lip
- Michael J. Fox, actor, Parkinson Disease
- Dustin Hoffman, actor, ADHD
- Leonardo DiCaprio, actor, obsessive compulsive disorder
- Heather Whitestone McCallum, Miss America queen, deaf
- Jessie Jackson, activist, cleft lip
- Jay Leno, TV host and comedian, dyslexia
- Tom Whittaker, amputee, reached the Mt. Everest summit
- Marlee Martin, actor, deaf

## Problem Solving

When problem solving, get the facts, talk to the experts, analyze, and review the plus/minuses of the decision. If something just doesn't add up, trust your intuition.

*Bernadette S.*

### Every Day

Don't become stagnate. Challenge yourself to learn, grow each day. Be open and honest with the people you meet.

*Joan H.*

### Money

Have your money work as hard as you do. Eliminate credit cards and high interest loans. If you are behind on loans, catch up as quickly as possible and then learn how to avid that problem. Learn about money and how to use it wisely.

*Jasmine W., advice from her mother*

### Short & Simple

KISS--Keep it simple, stupid

*Jennifer T.*

### Bank

Life is like a bank. You can withdraw thing from it, but you must pay it back. Take out what you need and leave some for others. Don't be greedy.

*Sandy K.*

### Decisions

This is not the last decision you will ever make. Once made, let it go.

*Amal H.*

## Accept Change

You can never dip your toe in the same spot in the river. Life is a series of twist and turns. Be able to make the flow work for you. Know when to be strong and when to be flexible.

*Sandra J.*

## Before the Job Interview

Separate yourself from the others looking for a job. Before an interview do some research on the company, the person who will be interviewing you and the industry. Ask good questions. Be prepared for the questions you will likely be asked.

*Vera D.*

## Care About People

When you are the boss, first care about your people, then lead them.

*Melissa L.*

## Don't Wait

"Don't wait; the time will never be just right."

*Keshon M., submitted this quote from Napoleon Hill, author of "Think and Grow Rich"*

## Easier to Remember

"Always tell the truth. It is the easiest to remember."

*Shandra P., submitted this quote from David Mamet*

### Encourage/Motivate

- Treat others the way that you would want to be treated.
- Manage as you would want to be managed. Motivate others as you would want to be motivated.
- Build your team on mutual respect.

*Maddi E., advice from her boss when she started managing people*

### Staying Employable

Regardless of your age, stay current. Read, take classes, network with others in the field, and get on industry committees. Network often. Let others in the industry know who you are.

*Monica F., advice from a career counselor*

## {QUOTE FOR DISCUSSION}

### His Credo

"The only true disability in life is a bad attitude."

*Scott Hamilton, Olympic Champion, cancer survivor from an article in AARP Magazine*

How does this quote relate to your life or someone you know? Do you have a bad attitude about your job, relationships, money, or the future?

_____
_____

## Break It

If it doesn't work, break it! Don't let someone who isn't growing stop you from advancing.

*Danelle R., advice for her Grandfather*

## Networking

Network as a giver, not as a taker. You will be rewarded.

*Jane G.*

## Attitude and Approach

What matters is your attitude and approach. Be open to new possibilities. Be ready for new opportunities you may never have thought of before.

*Gabriel A.*

## People

Be kind and caring to those you meet.

*Milli H.*

### Inspection
Always inspect what you expect.

*Stephanie S.*

### Humor
Don't lose your sense of humor.

*Valentina C., advice from her college advisor*

### Know Who You Are Dealing With
Don't throw pearls to a swine.

*Isabella D., advice from her Dad*

### Aim
If you aim at nothing you will hit it every time.

*Darlene W.*

### Learn to Respect
Everyone has their unique story. Learn to respect others. Kindness and empathy will help you throughout your life.

*June Z.*

# CHEROKEE INDIAN FOLKLORE

### Two Wolves

One evening an old Cherokee told his grandson about a battle that goes on inside people. He said, "My son, the battle is between two "wolves" inside us all.

### One wolf is EVIL

It is anger, envy, jealously, sorrow, regret, greed, arrogance, self-pity, guilt, resentment, inferiority, lies, false pride, and ego.

### The other is GOOD

It is joy, peace, love, hope, serenity, humility, kindness, empathy, generosity, truth, and faith.

The grandson thought for a minute and then asked his grandfather: "Which wolf will win?"

The old Cherokee simply replied, "The one you feed."

### Discussion Questions:

Do you know someone who is feeds the Evil wolf?

Which wolf do you feed?

_____
_____
_____
_____
_____
_____
_____
_____
_____
_____
_____
_____
_____

## Face Your Fears

Face your fears. Everyone has them. In a confrontation, the person who is the loudest or most boastful is usually the most scared. Conquer your fears.

*Emma J., advice from her martial arts instructor*

## Don't Borrow Money

When you owe money to people, credit cards or banks, you are basically working for them until the debt is repaid. Work for yourself not them.

*Liz S., advice from a money counselor*

## Procrastination

Don't procrastinate. Tackle the things you don't want to do first. Then the rest is easy. If you must do something, get on with it. When completed you can relax and take a well-deserved break.

*Janell Z.*

## Work for a Reason

Don't work just for the money. Find purpose. Continuous learning on and off the job.

*Iva B.*

## Your Ego

Don't let your ego spend money you don't have. (i.e., bigger house, faster car, or various status symbols)

*Joanna P.*

## Learn People Skills

People can be funny, kind, selfish, thoughtful, extroverted, caring, mean, thoughtless, stupid, egotistical, and more. But, unless you are going to be a hermit, you need to learn how to get along with all types. It will be more rewarding than frustrating – I promise.

*Janel L., advice from her mother*

## Size of the Dog

It's not the size of the dog, it's the size of the fight within the dog.

*Mae T.*

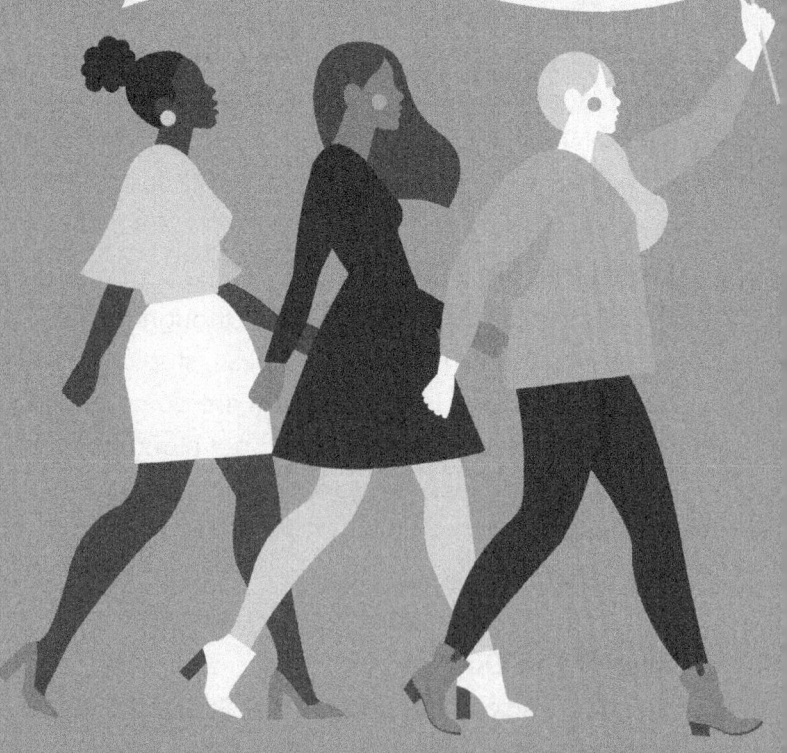

# 10 WAYS TO PREPARE FOR SUCCESS

Success takes time, planning, and a strong desire. Success means developing a plan and accomplishing your goals. Success is taking action - even when the going gets tough. Here are a few ideas to help develop a solid personal foundation to build on for your success.

1. **Education**
   - The importance of education cannot be overstated. It does not stop when you leave school. Become a continuous learner. Read more, ask questions, and listen. Find a mentor to help you.

2. **Skills**
   - Take a realistic inventory of your strengths and areas that need improvement. What do you like to do? What area do you want to improve and why?

3. **Develop a Plan**
   - Answer these questions: What do I want? How will I get it? When do I want it?
   - Write down a plan for your success that includes goals, individual action steps, and a timetable for completion.

4. **Find Inspiration**
   - You do not have to work alone. Find a role model or mentor who can be your trusted advisor. Find someone who has the experience and knowledge to guide you. Surround yourself with people who can help you reach your goals.

5. **Exceed Expectations**
   - Be determined, dependable and responsible. Be accountable for your words and actions. Become the "go-to" person in your group.

6. **Set Realistic Goals**
   - Set and achieve goals that will stretch your capabilities. Then, build on your successes. Reward yourself after you reach each goal.

7. **Use Your Time Wisely**
   - Manage your time or be mismanaged by it.

8. **Helping Others**
   - Twain once stated: "Kindness is the language which the deaf can hear and the blind can see." Successful people know the importance of helping others.

9. **Offer Solutions**
   - Don't find fault; find a solution. Separate yourself from those who make excuses, complain, or are judgmental of others. If you make a mistake, turn it into a learning exercise.

### 10. Maintain a Positive Attitude
- Believe in yourself, visualize your future success. Smile often. Develop a can-do attitude. Success breeds success.
- With these tools you will develop a solid financial foundation for your future growth.

**Suggestions for implementation:**
- Write down the two on this list that you do well. Be specific.
- Write the two items that are not your strong suit.
- Which item on the list do you want to focus on improving. It can be any of the ten.

_____
_____
_____
_____
_____
_____
_____
_____
_____
_____
_____
_____

## Leadership

Everything rises and falls on leadership.

*Adella M., advice quoted from John Maxwell*

## Forward Thinking

Don't do something that you will be embarrassed about tomorrow. When you look at yourself in the morning will you be ok with the image you see? Remorse is a bitter pill.

*Kathryn V.*

## Your Boss

Do all you can to keep your Boss's Boss off your Boss's Back!

*Darci U., advice from a HR Manager*

## Substituting for Adults

I tell students you can't solve adult problems. When adults are acting stupid or hurting themselves (i.e., drug or alcohol issues) they are often not listening to anyone. Find someone you can count on to help you. Get into a support group.

*Candence L., middle school teacher*

## College After High School

I meet countless people who wished they had gone to college when they were younger, before family, home, and responsibilities came into the picture. If you take a gap year stay focused on the prize.

*Nicole R.*

### Your Goals
Write down your goals. You cannot achieve what you can't not name.

*Phyllis P.*

## {QUOTE FOR DISCUSSION}

"You gain strength, courage, and confidence by every experience in which you really stop to look fear in the face."

*Eleanor Roosevelt*

Do you agree? Do you have a personal example of when you faced fear head on?

_____
_____
_____
_____
_____
_____

### Success' Intersection
Success is the intersection of desire, planning, determination, and focus. Helping others is always part of the equation.

*Simone J.*

### Every Successful Person
Do you define yourself by a failure? Have others moved on, but you're still stuck in the past? Every

person on Earth has failed, but some are much better and putting those negative experiences in the rear view mirror. Learn from the mistake or failure and silently say "Thank You", and then move on.

*Laurie H.*

Your thoughts?

_____
_____
_____
_____
_____
_____
_____
_____
_____
_____
_____
_____

## The Right Thing

Sometimes doing the right thing is the hardest thing in the world to do. Often your reward is knowing that you did it. Many will notice if you did it the wrong way. Few will notice when you did it in the right way.

*Iva B.*

## Television
Don't live life on a couch watching TV or a cellphone screen. Get out and try something knew even if t's hard at first.  You won't meet the person who can change your life watching TV. Get involved.

*Bella I.*

## Courage
Have courage and don't let everything get to you.

*Darcy V.*

## Alice in Wonderland
If you don't know where you are going, any road will get you there!

*Yvonne Y., advice from Alice in Wonderland*

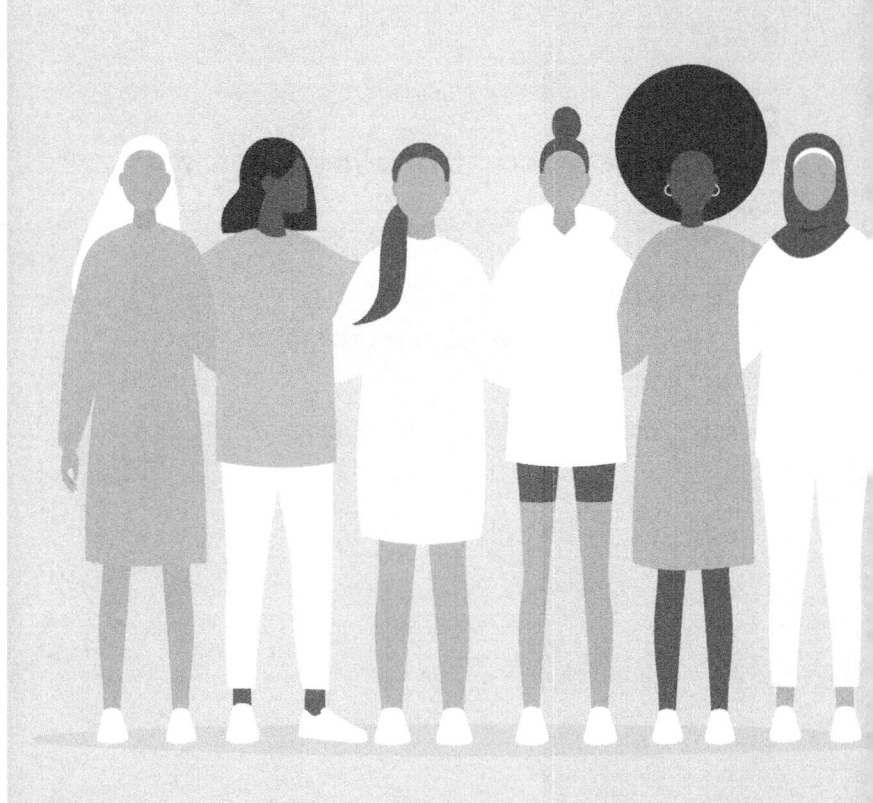

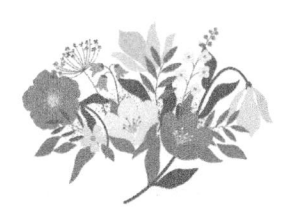

# ADVICE FROM OTHER CULTURES

Bruce Lee, the world-famous martial artist, told this story about his teacher as a lesson for one of his students. It is about the Japanese Zen master who received a university professor who came to inquire about Zen.

It was obvious that the professor from the start was not so much interested in learning about Zen as he was in impressing the master with his opinions and knowledge. The master listened patiently and finally suggested they have tea. The master poured the visitor's cup full and then kept pouring.

The professor watched the cup overflowing until he could no longer take it. "The cup is overfull, no more will go in." "Like this cup," the master said, "you are full of your own opinions and speculations. How can I show you Zen unless you first empty your cup?"

Bruce studied the student's face. "You understand the point?" "Yes," said the student, "You want me to empty my mind of past knowledge and old habits so that I will be open to new learning."

"Precisely," said Bruce Lee. "And now we are ready for the first lesson."

*Excerpt from Zen in the Martial Arts by Joe Hyams*

Your thoughts? Have you been close minded to new ideas?

_____
_____
_____
_____
_____
_____
_____
_____
_____
_____
_____
_____
_____
_____
_____
_____

### No vs. Yes

Don't accept NO from somebody who can't say YES!

*Nicci C., advice from a sales manager*

## Managing People

As a manager, surround yourself with the smart people, give them direction and a purpose, then get out of the way.

*Tamika H., advice from her boss*

## Time for Yourself

Whatever you do, make sure you make time for yourself.

*Yesha S., advice from a relative*

## Yourself

Don't take yourself too seriously.

*Regina R., advice from her Mom*

## Bridges

Don't burn bridges if you can't swim.

*Beth J.*

## LICENSE PLATE IDEA

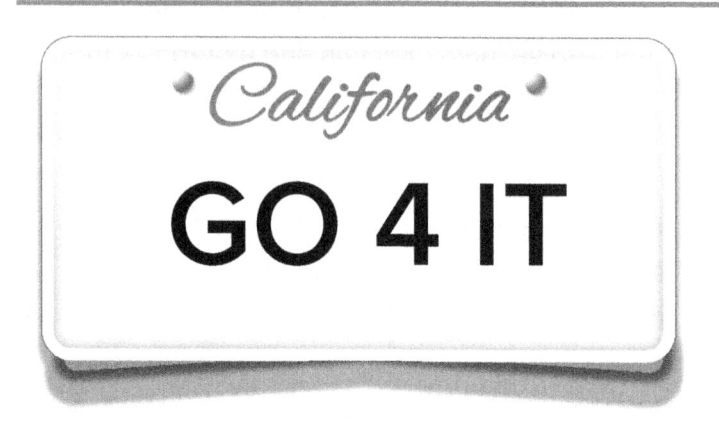

**GO 4 IT** (California)

The license plate will be a daily reminder for you, and it may help others.

### Doubt
When in doubt throw it out.

*Iris S.*

### Great Habits
Successful people have great habits that failures never do!

*Laqueta P.*

### Chronic Illness
To live well with a chronic illness is largely a mind game....Think about who you are and how you want to live. How will you make the most out of your life now? Do not stifle your dreams....

*Richard Cohen, writing about living with his chronic illness in AARP Magazine*

*Your thoughts?*

## Speak Up - Shut Up

Know when to speak up and know when to shut up. You'll be respected more and get into less trouble.

*Tanisha G.*

## Expectations

Managing your expectations. Rome was not built in a day.

*Samantha Z., advice from a teacher*

## Do It Well

Do more than you are asked. Do all jobs - big or small - well or not at all.

*Olivia F.*

# { QUOTE FOR DISCUSSION }

"To laugh often and much; to win the respect of intelligent people and the affection of children;...to appreciate beauty, to find the best in others; to leave the world a little better; whether by a healthy child or a garden patch....to know even one life has breathed easier because you have lived. This is success."

*Ralph Waldo Emerson*

Do you share Emerson's view of success? How do you define success?

_____
_____
_____
_____
_____
_____
_____
_____
_____
_____
_____
_____

## Have It All

Yes, you can have it all. Just remember to be grateful and share.

*Susan B.*

## Pennies are Important

Watch your pennies and the dollars will take care of themselves.

*Maria, T.*

## Stop Selling

Stop selling and start building relationships. Good advice in sales and in life.

*Danelle C.*

## Managing Your Boss

Never care about a project more than your boss. Make her look good to her boss.

*Tyesha S., advice from a mentor*

## Excuses

Your problems, are they your excuse or your motivation?

*Johanna N.*

## Ask Questions

The only "stupid" question is the one you don't ask.

*Lilly S.*

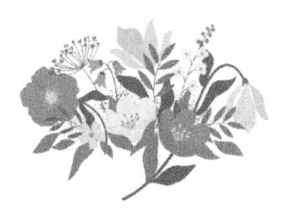

# 10 RULES ABOUT MONEY

How we view money has a profound impact on all facets of our life. It determines where we live, the type of job we have, how we look at the world, and, unfortunately, how we feel about ourselves. Money has the power to do great things, but it can also destroy the mightiest empires.

Each of us must determine what our relationship with money will be. We must learn how to earn it, save it, spend it, and invest it. These can be hard lessons, but you can use a few simple rules to make your life a lot less stressful.

1. Control your spending or it will control you.
2. Work smart for your money.
3. With savings and investments, have your money work as hard as you do.
4. Minimize or eliminate high-interest debt (i.e., credit cards, rent to own, payday loans, buy now/pay later loans, etc.).
5. Surround yourself with people who know how to use money wisely.
6. Put at least 5% from every paycheck into a savings account.

7. Do not let money determine your self-image.
8. If your company has automatic deposit for your paycheck, use it.
9. Remember: It is not how much you earn; it is how much you keep that counts.
10. To earn more—learn more, do more and think more.

Follow these rules and money issues will work in your favor rather than against you.

**Suggestions for Implementation:**

1. Find a mentor who can teach you about the fundamentals of money.
2. Have open family discussions about money.
3. Think of your last major purchase. Did you really need the item? Or did you simply want it?

How many of the 10 Rules on Money are currently doing well? Which two rules to you need to work on in the next six months?

_____
_____
_____
_____
_____
_____
_____
_____

## How You Get It
Education is expensive.... no matter how you get it.
*Laqueta C.*

## Begin
Begin with a clear view of the prize. Finish strong.
*Carmen O.*

## Helping Others
Helping others helps you. Treat all people with respect.
*Keshon A.*

## What They Need
Give customers what they asked for, and then give them what they need.
*Charlotte Z.*

## Have a Goal
Have a goal in life. Lots of people are simply going through the motions. Read, ask questions, be realistic and reward yourself when you reach your goal.
*Candi W.*

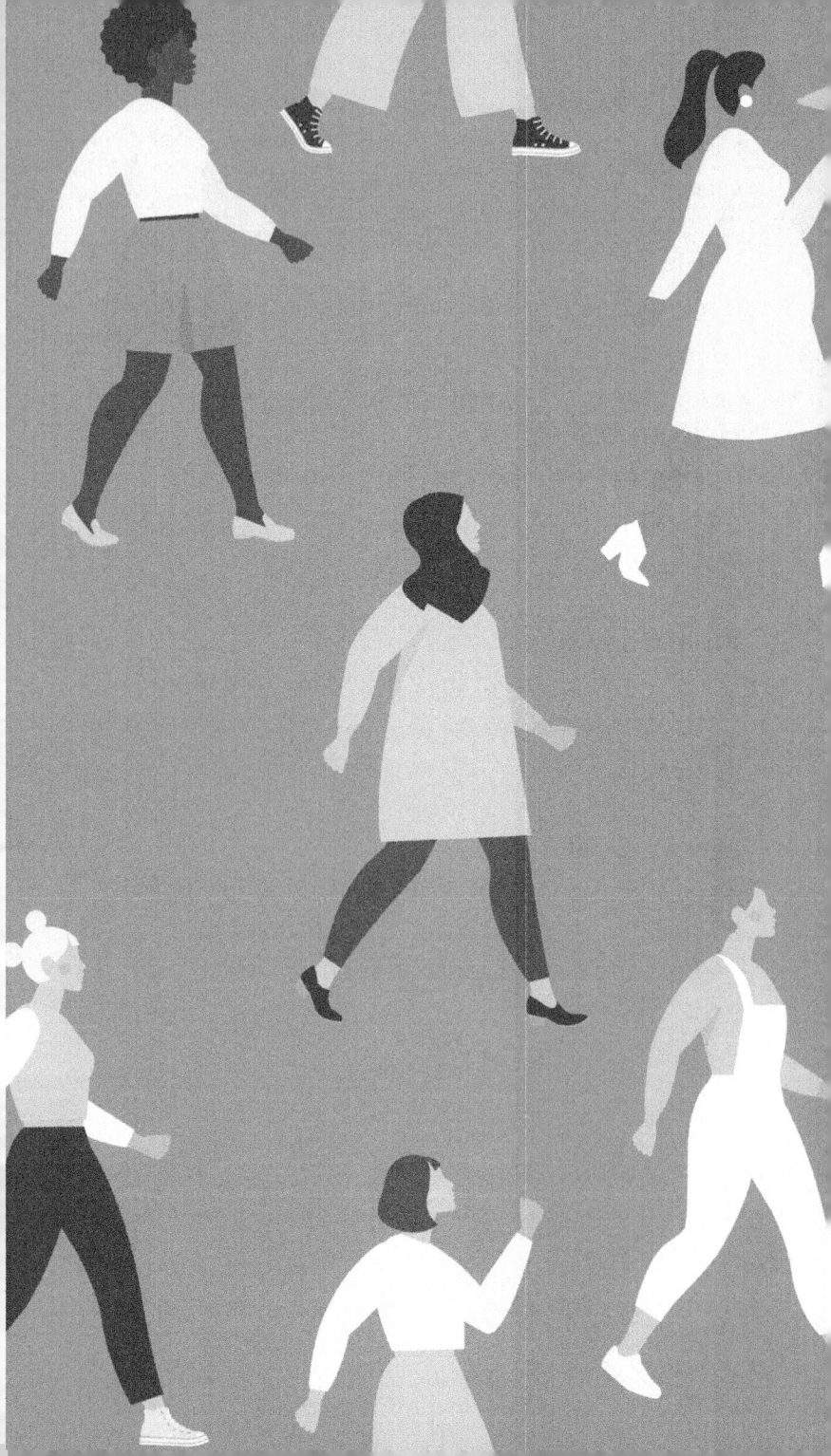

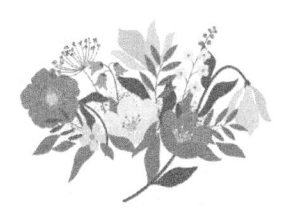

# YOU ARE NOT ALONE

**Famous people who have overcome disabilities**

- Billy Joel, songwriter, singer, depression
- Terry Fox, humanitarian, amputee, ran across Canada to raise funds for cancer research
- Muhammad Ali, boxer, Parkinson Disease
- Brenda Gildehaus, BMX rider, multiple sclerosis
- Montel Williams, TV talk show host, multiple sclerosis
- Stephen Hawking, scientist, Lou Gehrig's disease (ALS)
- Teddy Roosevelt, U.S. President, epilepsy
- John Cougar Mellencamp, singer, Spina Bifida
- Cheech Martin, actor, cleft lip
- Magic Johnson, NBA star, ADHD, AIDS

## Your Resume

Make sure you have a new line in your resume each year. Accomplishments matter.

Teamwork matters more.

*Adrian H.*

### Energize Yourself

In this hectic, puzzling world, don't forget to take time for yourself. Go to a concert, read a book, go for a walk, go camping. Recharging your batteries will give you a fresh perspective on life.

*Estelle V , advice from her friend*

### Double Check

Double check EVERYTHING before you pull the trigger.

*Johanna A.*

### Perfection

Don't let the perfect be the enemy of the good.

*Jennifer A., submitted this quote from Voltaire*

### Email

Never check email before 10:00 am. This is the title to a book, and its great idea.

*Peggy J.*

### Emotional Quotient

Sometimes you simply must agree to disagree. You'll be greatly disappointed if you try to win every argument.

*Kamilla Q.*

### Breathing

Take deep breaths and smile. You can do this.

*Rachel C.*

**Eight Inches**

There's only eight inches between a pat on the back and a kick in the ass.

*Katie M.*

## LICENSE PLATE IDEA

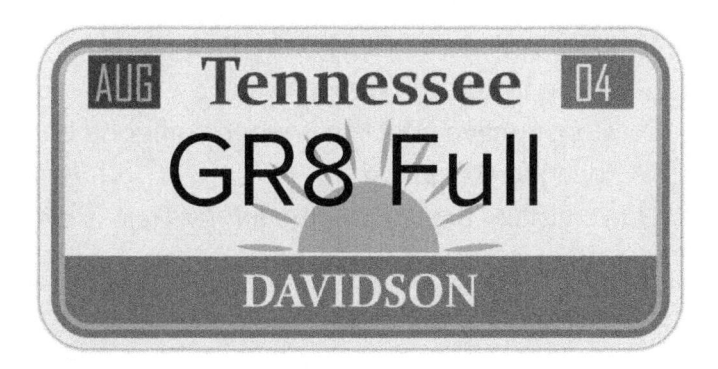

**AUG Tennessee 04**
**GR8 Full**
DAVIDSON

This will be a daily reminder for you,

and it may help others.

**Impossible**

Nothing is Impossible! Hard - yes. Impossible – never. About the time you think you can't, you''' find someone already doing it.

*Iva S.*

**New Experiences**

Treat each new experience as an opportunity to learn. The tougher it is the hard you must try. Each failure gets you that much closer to success.

*Susan K.*

## Activity

Doing busy work will not lead to accomplishments. Stay focused on how each step gets you closer to your goal.

*Patricia O.*

## Criticism

There are two types of criticism.

1. Destructive criticism is when someone is trying to put you down.
2. Constructive criticism is when someone is trying to lift you up.

Don't mistake the later for the former. Help is everywhere if you are receptive.

*Regina R.*

## Find Answers

Be inquisitive. Learn to question anything and learn to find answer on your own.

*Amelia O.*

## Before

Do what you have to do BEFORE you do what you want to do.

*Tyesha J.*

# 10 LIFE LESSONS LEARNED ON A UNICYCLE

Ever try to ride a unicycle? Many people call it "terror on a stick," and I agree. But it is also a great teacher of some valuable life lessons.

My husband chose a unicycle to teach our grandchildren a valuable lesson. At sixty years old, many of my friends thought John was out of my mind. In truth, I thought they were right. But he felt it was important to teach my grandchildren them about determination, extra effort and getting up after a fall. Riding a unicycle is not easy at any age, but at sixty it was a real eye-opener.

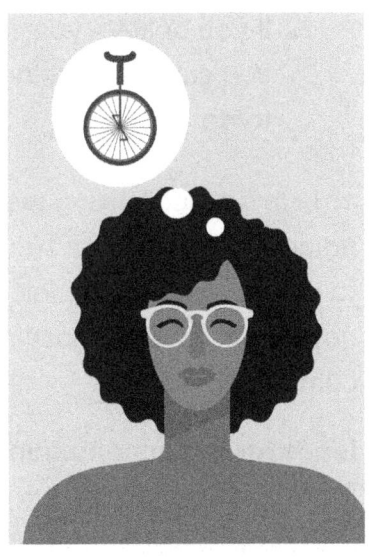

**10 Life Lessons Learned on a Unicycle:**

- •Some of life's lessons are painful but keep

trying.
- Determination helps you overcome your fears.
- You will not go far without balance in your life.
- Breathe naturally, even when you are afraid.
- Practice, practice, practice.
- Do not be concerned about what others are saying.
- On a unicycle you will stand out in a crowd.
- You are as old as you think you are.
- If you believe you can - go for it.
- You can do anything you make your mind up to do.

I am not suggesting that everyone should start riding a unicycle. I am suggesting that it is important to get out of your comfort zone and try something new. Some of life's most important lessons do not come easy.

**Ideas for Implementation**

What have you always wanted to do? Take singing lessons, hike the Appalachian Trail, or take a college course?

_____
_____
_____
_____
_____
_____
_____

## People and Book Covers
Be respectful and inclusive of all people. Don't judge a book by its cover. This is nothing new but is so true.

*Janell Z.*

## Loving It
Do what you love. It sounds simple but it is the truth.

*Stefani B.*

## 5 Second Decisions
The most important life changing decisions you will make as a teen will take 5 seconds. Should I get in that car? Should I leave this party? Should I try a cigarette? Those decisions take 5 seconds, but they can profoundly affect the rest of your life.

*Karen A, advice for her college daughter*

## Promise vs. Deliver
Under promise. Over deliver.

*Jessie N.*

## After You Know Everything
It's what you learn after you think you know everything that's important.

*Jessi A., advice from her father*

## Value

Always add value!

*Stefanie K.*

## Judgment

Judge not, or you will be judged.

*Lillian D.*

## Your Turn

What 3 things from the Empowered Women Helping Others book do you want to incorporate into your everyday life?

_____
_____
_____
_____
_____
_____
_____

# What Have You Learned About Yourself?

## AUTHORS BIOGRAPHIES

John and I are passionate about two things:

1. More women should be in positions of power.

2. We want our grandchildren to live in a world that embraces strong American values – that are equally accessible to everyone.

Carole has over twenty-five years of experience in counseling, specializing in women's issues, grief work and life coaching. In the corporate world, her expertise includes executive coaching, motivation, training, conflict resolution and employee selection.

John has owned two companies and was the VP – Sales in another company with 300 salespeople. In his free time, he has camped alone at the bottom of the Grand Canyon for seven days and earned two black belts in Martial Arts.

Their focus is on helping people succeed. Together, they have owned a management consulting business for over twenty-five years working with companies on selection, retention, and engagement issues. Personally, they are blessed with two daughters and seven grandchildren.

Made in the USA
Las Vegas, NV
21 May 2021